Six-Minute Social Skills - 3

Friendship Skills for Kids with Autism & Asperger's

Janine Toole PhD

Happy Frog Learning

Happy Frog Learning

www.HappyFrogLearning.com

About Happy Frog Learning

Happy Frog Learning creates high-quality resources for elementary and high school children with autism and other social/language challenges.

We believe that all children can learn – as long as we provide a learning environment that suits their needs.

www.HappyFrogLearning.com

Friendship Skills for Kids with Autism & Asperger's

Table of Contents

Introduction: Six-Minute Social Skills 1

Chapter 1 What Is A Friend? 9

    1.1 Friends are fun 11

    1.2 Friends accept each other 13

    1.3 Friends share interests 15

    1.4 Friends are kind 17

    1.5 Friends do things together 19

    1.6 Friends listen to each other 21

    1.7 Friendship is a choice between two people 23

Chapter 2 Building a Friendship 25

    2.1 Pay attention 27

    2.2 Ask questions 29

    2.3 Choose topics of interest 31

    2.4 Body orientation 33

    2.5 Read faces 35

    2.6 Space invader 37

    2.7 Make decisions together 39

    2.8 Compromise 41

    2.9 Not my choice 43

    2.10 Be a good sport 45

    2.11 Friends share 47

Chapter 3 When Things Go Wrong 49

    3.1 Consider my own behavior 51

    3.2 Apologize if needed 53

    3.3 State my problem 55

3.4 Choose something else..57

3.5 Accept other's opinions...59

3.6 Cool down...61

3.7 No hard feelings..63

Chapter 4 Challenging Situations...65

4.1 Saying no 67

4.2 Suggest an alternative..69

4.3 Walk away 71

4.4 Talk to an adult 73

4.5 False friends...75

Chapter 5 Fun Things to do with Friends 77

5.1 Activity Evaluation: Active Structured Play 81

5.2 Activity Evaluation: Active Unstructured Play...83

5.3 Activity Evaluation: Board Games & Card Games 85

5.4 Activity Evaluation: Video Games...87

5.5 Activity Evaluation: Building & Creating 89

5.6 Activity Evaluation: Comparing Thoughts & Opinions.............................91

5.7 Activity Evaluation: Talking about Shared Experiences 93

5.8 Activity Evaluation: Making Plans...95

5.9 Activity Evaluation: 96

Introduction: Six-Minute Social Skills

Welcome to the *Six-Minute Social Skills* series. This series is designed for busy parents and professionals who need easy-to-use and effective materials to work with learners who have Autism, Asperger's and similar social skill challenges.

This workbook, *Friendship Skills,* provides step-by-step activities to quickly build social confidence. With the clear and easy-to-use worksheets, your student will learn:

- What a friend is... and how to recognize what friendship looks like

- How to show friendship with your actions and words

- How to build a friendship through sharing activities and interests

- What to do when things go wrong so you can get your friendship back on track

- How to recognize and deal with false friends.

These skills are developed incrementally, with lots of practice, allowing your learner to make meaningful progress week by week.

The workbook contains forty worksheets, organized into five chapters. Each worksheet is preceded by a parent/educator guide containing suggestions for alternate and extension activities.

Children with ASD need practice at developing their friendship skills. With this workbook, you can ensure they have the tools to build and maintain enduring friendships.

Key Ideas Summary

Download a one-page summary of all the Key Ideas

introduced in the workbook. Great for quick reference!

Available for free on our website:

www.HappyFrogLearning.com/Friendship-Skills-PDF

Don't forget to check out the other books in our Six-Minute Social Skills series. Although numbered, the books can be used in any order.

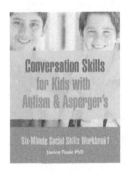
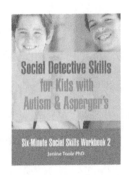

Available in print or Kindle

on Amazon

How to Coach a Six-Minute Session

We want you and your learner to have fun when you coach a six-minute session. So here are some suggestions.

1. Don't worry if you never write in the workbook!

Filling in a workbook is NOT practicing friendship skills. What's most important is discussing the ideas and examples that are contained in each worksheet and doing role-plays, when appropriate.

So use the workbook as you need. Use it as a guide for discussion, a guide for oral practice and role-plays, or as an actual worksheet... whatever helps your student learn something new.

2. Don't be afraid to repeat.

In the six-minute series, we have broken down social skills into tiny steps. But even so, your learner will not develop these skills instantly. Don't be afraid to repeat a worksheet until your learner develops confidence.

If you are concerned about boredom, mix your review in with new lessons. In any case, don't move too far ahead if your learner still needs help with earlier skills.

3. Make sure to reciprocate.

A great way to learn is to be the teacher. Once your learner shows progress at a skill, switch the roles so that **you** have to reply to a situation or problem that they pose to you. Periodically, make an error and get your learner to tell you what's wrong with your response.

4. Have a consistent schedule.

Consistency is important if you want to reach a goal. Choose a regular schedule for your six-minute sessions. Get your learner's agreement and stick to it!

We also recommend having a consistent method for delivering each six-minute session. This allows you to move quickly and helps your learner stay focused. Here's a schedule we have found successful.

1. Review the last lesson

Briefly review the Key Idea and activity from the most recent worksheet. Allow the student to see the worksheet as you discuss it.

> *Let's get started. Here's what we did last time. Do you remember what the Key Idea was for that lesson?*
>
> *<wait for student response>*
>
> *Right. And what did this diagram show?*
>
> *<wait for student response>*
>
> *Awesome. Let's see what we do today.*

2. Introduce today's Key Idea

All lessons have a Key Idea. This is a simple 'social rule' that is vital for students to know. Once you have introduced a Key Idea, you can reference it when needed during everyday life.

For example, once you have introduced the key idea that everyone in a situation has social expectations, you can remind your learner when he or she considers only his/her own interests.

During a lesson, use a 3-step process to introduce the Key Idea.

1. READ:

Get your learner to read the key idea or read it for your student if reading is a challenge.

> *Here is today's key idea. Can you read it for me?*

2. PARAPHRASE:

After the student has read the key idea, briefly paraphrase it in a way that is sensitive to your student's comprehension level and makes it more relevant to their experiences.

> *Good reading! So, I guess that is saying that everyone in a situation has their own thoughts about how everyone should behave.*

3. CONNECT:

Talk with your learner about the key idea. Can they think of any examples in their life where the key idea is relevant?

3. Complete & review the worksheet

You can fill in the worksheet by writing or complete the worksheet orally. Either approach is effective.

Provide the support your student needs to complete the worksheet. Keep in mind that your goal for every worksheet is for your learner to reach the point where they can independently demonstrate an understanding of the social rule, both during your six-minute sessions and in actual real-life situations.

Once the worksheet is complete, review it together. If your student finds this difficult, you can provide a model. Describe or paraphrase what the student has written/said. Where possible, relate it back to the key idea. For example:

> *I see that you noted that one of your expectations when you watch TV is that no one will change the channel without asking.*
>
> *That's a reasonable expectation. I have that expectation too.*

4. Extra practice (optional)

Your learner may need extra practice. Most worksheets have suggestions for how to extend the skill development.

5. Revisit the Key Idea

To finish up, draw your learner's attention back to the Key Idea. Ask them to tell you the key idea and then ask your student a question that relates the key idea to the worksheet or to the student's life.

> *Nice job. Now let's look at the Key Idea again. What was our Key Idea?*
>
> *<wait for student response>*
>
> *Yes. We all have expectations about how everyone will behave. Can you think of an expectation I might have if I am talking on the phone?*
>
> *<wait for student response>*

Fantastic! Yes, my expectation is that I won't be interrupted unless it is really important.

6. Congratulate your learner & finish

You should provide encouraging feedback throughout the six-minute session. Make sure to also finish up on a positive note. Congratulate your student and identify something they did well during the session.

Most of all, don't forget to have fun!

Chapter 1
What Is A Friend?

Introduction

In this chapter we talk about what makes a good friend.

There are lots of nice people in the world, but not everyone is a good choice to be YOUR friend. Your friends will be people that are a good match for you – and you are a good match for them!

Let's find out how to tell whether someone is a good friend match for you.

1.1 Coaching Guide: Friends are fun

Quick Reference:

» Introduce the 'Six-Minute Social Skills' workbook

» Introduce the Key Idea: Read, paraphrase, connect

» Complete & review the worksheet

» Extra practice

» Revisit the Key Idea

» Congratulate your learner & finish

General Notes: The goal of this worksheet is to introduce the central idea that friends should be fun to be with. Right from the start, we also want to emphasize that what is fun for one person, may not be enjoyable for another person. Each child needs to look for friends that suit him or her.

Extra Practice: Talk about peers that your child knows and identify which ones your child enjoys being with. Ask why they enjoy being with that peer. Be open to hearing about peers that your learner does not find fun. Again, ask questions to find out why.

Your Notes/Extra Ideas:

1.1 Friends are fun

Key  *Idea*

A friend is fun to hang out with and play with.

I enjoy myself when I spend time with a friend.

Joe is a very active 9-year-old who wants to hang out with someone at lunchtime. Who is he more likely to have fun with? Why?

- Kiera likes to sit near the playground and make daisy chains with friends.

- Liam brings a basketball to school every day and is always looking for someone to play ball with.

- Jack loves the swings. He goes on the swings for the whole lunchtime.

Mia is new and she is trying to decide which lunch club to join. She likes doing puzzles and playing strategy games. Where is she most likely to have fun? Where is she most likely to make friends?

- Chess Club
- Yarn Club
- Sports Club

1.2 Coaching Guide: Friends accept each other

Quick Reference:

» Review the last worksheet

» Introduce the Key Idea: Read, paraphrase, connect

» Complete & review the worksheet

» Extra practice

» Revisit the Key Idea

» Congratulate your learner & finish

General Notes: Children with ASD are often aware that they are different from other children. The purpose of this worksheet is to reinforce that a good friend is happy with us as we are. We don't need to change or be someone different with a true friend.

An additional note: In this worksheet, and others throughout the book, we ask about who would make a good friend choice. The purpose is NOT to separate peers into 'good' friend choices and 'bad' friend choices. Rather, it is to help our learners start thinking about what they have in common with friends and who they like to spend time with. Please make sure your learner doesn't slip into black and white thinking about who is a good friend and who is not.

Extra Practice: Depending on the age and awareness of your learner, consider asking if they have sometimes tried to be different in order to fit in, or if they feel more comfortable with being themselves in some situations over others.

Your Notes/Extra Ideas:

1.2 Friends accept each other

A friend accepts me as I am.

Consider these situations.

Kian needs to hum quietly as he works. It helps him concentrate. Frank sits behind Kian and finds the humming annoying. Frank always gives an exasperated sigh when he hears the humming.   Joe sits right next to Kian and doesn't seem to notice the humming.

    1. Which student accepts Kian as he is?

    2. Who is a better choice for a friend? Why?

_____

_____

Joe sometimes takes a while to explain things. His friends Matt always jumps in and explains things for him, even when Joe doesn't want him to. His other friend Pietro just lets Joe take his time.

    1. Which friend accepts Joe as he is?

    2. How can Matt be a better friend to Joe?

_____

_____

1.3 Coaching Guide: Friends Share Interests

Quick Reference:

» Review the last worksheet

» Introduce the Key Idea: Read, paraphrase, connect

» Complete & review the worksheet

» Extra practice

» Revisit the Key Idea

» Congratulate your learner & finish

General Notes: A key part of friendship is doing fun activities together. So, a basic requirement for a good friend is that they enjoy doing some of the same things. The most available peer might be an awesome kid, but if he and your learner don't have some shared interests, it will be difficult for the friendship to flourish.

When completing the worksheet with your learner, find lots of connections between the children mentioned. Interests don't have to be exactly the same for a strong connection. For example, a soccer player will probably get on with any active kid. A student who loves roller coasters may connect with a learner who likes building things, including roller coasters, etc.

Making these varied connections may help your learner make connections from their own narrow interests to other possibilities.

Extra Practice: Get your learner to think about the things that he or she likes to do. Now compare those preferences to your learner's peers to see where the strong matches are. Consider also where else peers with this interest might be found. Think widely about relevant special interest groups, community groups, etc.

Your Notes/Extra Ideas:

1.3 Friends share interests

Friends enjoy many of the same activities.

Identify the kids who are more likely to be friends.

Abby loves skiing and reading.

Bert wants to be a geologist.

Carla has lots of energy and loves active play.

Dave loves building things out of anything.

Elsie likes cooking but hates reading.

Fiona hates the cold and prefers to read science books.

Greg loves roller coasters and eating at restaurants.

Hugh wants to learn to snowboard and has three cats.

Jessi loves soccer and eating unusual food.

Karl spends all day drawing.

Luanne loves collecting things.

Martin loves sewing costumes and singing.

Nia wants to start a dog walking business.

Olli loves math puzzles and digging for gold.

Pietra plays role-playing games.

Quincy listens to music all day.

1.4 Coaching Guide: Friends are kind

Quick Reference:

» Review the last worksheet

» Introduce the Key Idea: Read, paraphrase, connect

» Complete & review the worksheet

» Extra practice

» Revisit the Key Idea

» Congratulate your learner & finish

General Notes: Children with Autism are often targets for bullying by school peers. So, it is important for ASD kids to know that kindness is one of the basic requirements for friendship. If someone isn't being kind, they are not acting like a friend.

Extra Practice: Your student may also have some learning to do around being kind to other children. If appropriate, use this worksheet as an opportunity to talk about how your learner can act more like a friend.

Your Notes/Extra Ideas:

1.4 Friends are kind

Friends are kind to each other.

Consider these situations.

Vince is wearing a new T-shirt with his favorite cartoon character on it. During the day, two kids in his class comment on the shirt.

- Cool kid that everyone wants to hang out with: "Hey Vince, is that your little brother's shirt?"

- Quiet kid that Vince doesn't know very well: "Hey Vince, who's that on your shirt?"

Which student is being kinder? Who is a better choice for a friend?

_____

_____

Gina is walking with her class when she drops her pencil box in the school hallway. Pencils and crayons go everywhere. A girl named Sasha stops and helps her pick up everything. Another girl named Erin steps over the mess and keeps walking.

Which student is showing kindness? Who would be a better choice to be a friend?

_____

_____

1.5 Coaching Guide: Friends do things together

Quick Reference:

>> Review the last worksheet

>> Introduce the Key Idea: Read, paraphrase, connect

>> Complete & review the worksheet

>> Extra practice

>> Revisit the Key Idea

>> Congratulate your learner & finish

General Notes: Friendships are built through shared activities. i.e. by doing things together. Our ASD learners are sometimes loners, who don't quite understand that to call someone a friend, you need to choose to do things together.

Use this worksheet to help your learner understand that friendships are built and maintained by choosing to do things with our friends.

Extra Practice: If possible, talk about some of the peers in your learner's class or community. Which ones does your learner do things with? Which ones can be called good friends? Which ones would your learner like to build a friendship with? If your learner is ready or interested in building a better friendship with a particular peer, work with him or her to help make that happen.

Your Notes/Extra Ideas:

1.5 Friends do things together

Friends do things together.

Consider these situations.

Leslie calls Gina her best friend, even though they never play together. Leslie usually spends her time hanging out with the kids in the chess club.

Is Gina really Leslie's best friend? Who are more likely to be Leslie's friends?

_____

_____

Tom calls Otis his friend, but whenever Otis wants to play, Tom says no. He prefers to spend time by himself. He even refused to go to Otis's birthday party.

Otis and Tom are friendly to each other, but are they building a friendship? Why or why not?

_____

_____

Casey prefers to read books at lunchtime, but sometimes if her classmate Leeza asks her to play basketball she'll go and play for a while.

Are Casey and Leeza building a friendship? Why or why not?

_____

_____

1.6 Coaching Guide: Friends listen to each other

Quick Reference:

>> Review the last worksheet

>> Introduce the Key Idea: Read, paraphrase, connect

>> Complete & review the worksheet

>> Extra practice

>> Revisit the Key Idea

>> Congratulate your learner & finish

General Notes: As well as doing things together, building a friendship requires that we listen to each other.

The purpose of this worksheet it to help your learner understand that attending/listening is a large component of friendship. Our friends will listen to us, and we should listen to our friends. While it may be difficult, it must be done.

Extra Practice: Your learner may need targeted support in listening/attending to their friends. Consider using the first workbook in the Six-Minute Social Skills series to build their conversation and attending skills.

Your Notes/Extra Ideas:

1.6 Friends listen to each other

A friend listens to me, and I listen to him or her.

Read the following conversations and identify who is doing a good job of listening and who is not.

Arnie:	Did you watch the game on Sunday?
Jake:	Yeah. It was awesome. What did you think of that final goal?
BJ:	The water park opened this weekend. Did you guys go?

How do you think Jake feels about BJ changing the topic before anyone had answered his question? Is that good for a friendship?

_____

_____

Kayla:	My sister got engaged on the weekend.
Lisa:	Oh, really! That's so exciting!
Reilly:	When's the wedding?
Sienna:	I went shopping with my sister on Saturday.

How do you think the other girls felt about what Sienna said?

Is that good for a friendship?

_____

_____

1.7 Coaching Guide: Friendship is a choice between two people

Quick Reference:

» Review the last worksheet

» Introduce the Key Idea: Read, paraphrase, connect

» Complete & review the worksheet

» Extra practice

» Revisit the Key Idea

» Congratulate your learner & finish

General Notes: The purpose of this worksheet is to teach your learner that friendship is a choice between two people. Your learner may want to be a friend with someone, but that person may not want to pursue a friendship with your student. Help your learner understand that people are different in many ways and not everyone is suited to be friends with each other.

True friendship comes when both people want to be friends with each other.

Extra Practice: Talk to your learner about their experiences. Have they wished for a friendship that was not reciprocated? Have they avoided building a relationship with another peer?

Your Notes/Extra Ideas:

1.7 Friendship is a choice between two people

Friendship is a choice between two people.

Both people have to want to be friends with each other.

Consider these situations:

Melanie is having fun doing a group project with Kyla and Ria. When the bell rings for lunch, Melanie asks them if they want to have lunch with her. Here's what they each say.

Kyla: Thanks, but I've already made plans with my friends.

Ria: Sure. Can I invite Lisa, too?

What can you guess about each girl and their willingness to build a friendship with Melanie?

_____

_____

Jim wants to get to know Lucas better. He tries inviting Lucas over to his place a few times, but Lucas always seems to have something else on. Lucas is polite, but he doesn't suggest a different time to get together.

What can you guess about Lucas's willingness to build a friendship with Jim?

Is it okay for Lucas to feel like this?

_____

_____

Chapter 2
Building a Friendship

In order to build a friendship, you need to act like a friend. This involves showing interest, listening, making decisions together and lots of other little steps that show our friend that we like them and like doing things with them.

This chapter will show you step-by-step how to act like a friend and build a friendship.

2.1 Coaching Guide: Pay attention

Quick Reference:

> » Review the last worksheet

> » Introduce the Key Idea: Read, paraphrase, connect

> » Complete & review the worksheet

> » Extra practice

> » Revisit the Key Idea

> » Congratulate your learner & finish

General Notes: A key skill for friendship is to be able to attend to a friend's words and actions. To connect with a friend, your learner must first give their attention to the friend.

In this worksheet, your student learns that attention sends positive messages to a peer.

Extra Practice: If you have examples from your learner's experiences, discuss how they may have missed friendship overtures. Choose some typical peer activities and role-play them with your student. Give guidance/prompts on how to attend. The skill may not come easily to your learner, and he/she may need specific instruction.

Your Notes/Extra Ideas:

2.1 Pay attention

To show I am interested in being a friend,

I pay attention to what my friend is doing.

Paying attention means watching and listening to what your friend is doing. By paying attention, you are showing that you are interested in him or her.

Jake is building a tower and is looking for the perfect block to finish it off. Ben passes him a red block that matches the rest of the blocks at the top of the tower.

Situation 1:   Jake takes the block and says thanks.

Is Ben paying attention to Jake?_____

Is Jake paying attention to Ben?_____

Are they building a good friendship?_____

Situation 2: Jake doesn't notice that Ben is holding out a block and picks up a different one and puts it on the tower.

Is Ben paying attention to Jake?_____

Is Jake paying attention to Ben?_____

How might Ben feel about Jake ignoring him?_____

What does this mean for their friendship?_____

2.2 Coaching Guide: Ask questions

Quick Reference:

  » Review the last worksheet

  » Introduce the Key Idea: Read, paraphrase, connect

  » Complete & review the worksheet

  » Extra practice

  » Revisit the Key Idea

  » Congratulate your learner & finish

General Notes: This worksheet reinforces the premise of the previous worksheet, that we need to show interest in order to build a friendship. An easy way to show interest is to ask questions. In this lesson, your learner practices asking questions in order to show interest and learn more about his friend.

Extra Practice: Draw from situations and peers in your learner's life. Help your learner role-play ways of showing interest.

For more practice, get the first workbook in the Six-Minute Series, Conversation Skills for Kids with Autism & Asperger's.

Your Notes/Extra Ideas:

2.2 Ask questions

To show I am interested in building a friendship,

I ask questions.

Consider these situations.

Kasen comes to school very excited and shows you and some other kids a rock that his uncle gave him.

You like Kasen and would like to be his friend. What questions could you ask to show you are interested?

_____

_____

The girl next to you in art class has just finished her painting. What questions can you ask to show that you are interested?

_____

_____

The new boy is sitting by himself reading a book at lunch time. What questions could you ask to show you are interested?

_____

_____

2.3 Coaching Guide: Choose topics of interest

Quick Reference:

» Review the last worksheet

» Introduce the Key Idea: Read, paraphrase, connect

» Complete & review the worksheet

» Extra practice

» Revisit the Key Idea

» Congratulate your learner & finish

General Notes: The purpose of this worksheet is to ensure your learner knows that he must show interest in topics and activities that his peer is interested in. Talking about his own interests does not build a friendship.

Extra Practice: If you know your student's shortcomings on this topic, use them as role-play situations and get your learner to actually perform more appropriate friendship-building responses.

Your Notes/Extra Ideas:

2.3 Choose topics of interest

To show I am interested in being friends,

I talk about things my friend is interested in.

Consider these situations.

Greg and Jerry are waiting for class to start. Greg starts telling Jerry all about his trip to a theme park on the weekend. Jerry listens but doesn't get a chance to ask any questions because Greg just keeps telling him about all the rides he went on and the food he ate.

Is a friendship being built here? Why or why not?

_____

Role-play this situation with your coach. You be Greg. How can you re-do this scene so that your conversation actually builds a friendship between you and Jerry?

Henry is super excited about his new bicycle. He tells Ty that he got a new bike, but Ty just shrugs and goes back to eating his lunch.

Is a friendship being built here? Why or why not?

_____

Role-play this situation with your coach. You be Ty. How can you re-do this scene so that your conversation actually builds a friendship between you and Henry?

2.4 Coaching Guide: Body orientation

Quick Reference:

> » Review the last worksheet
>
> » Introduce the Key Idea: Read, paraphrase, connect
>
> » Complete & review the worksheet
>
> » Extra practice
>
> » Revisit the Key Idea
>
> » Congratulate your learner & finish

General Notes: The purpose of this worksheet is to make students aware that body position communicates information. Your learner should make sure that what they communicate matches their intentions.

Extra Practice: Role-play with your learner to practice both demonstrating and interpreting body position.

Your Notes/Extra Ideas:

2.4 Body orientation

To show I am interested in being friends,

I turn my body towards my friend.

It may seem crazy, but the direction of your face and body communicates information. Turn your body toward your friend to show interest.

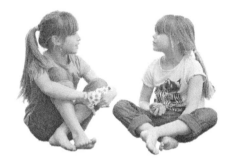

Are the girls showing interest in each other?

_____

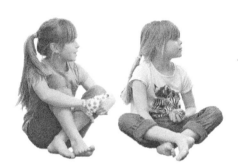

Are the girls showing interest in each other?

_____

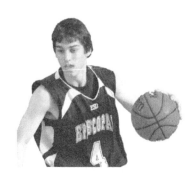

Peter is playing basketball by himself at the park. Joe would like to join in Peter's game. What can he do with his body to show interest?

_____

2.5 Coaching Guide: Read faces

Quick Reference:

> » Review the last worksheet

> » Introduce the Key Idea: Read, paraphrase, connect

> » Complete & review the worksheet

> » Extra practice

> » Revisit the Key Idea

> » Congratulate your learner & finish

General Notes: Eye contact is difficult for many children on the spectrum, so avoid targeting it as a specific goal. Instead, encourage learners to regularly check in with their friend's face so they don't miss important information.

Helping your learner understand why it is useful to check their friend's face, may give more motivation for this difficult task.

Extra Practice: Role-play situations from your student's daily life. Communicate key information without words so that your learner has to check in to know what is going on.

Your Notes/Extra Ideas:

2.5 Read faces

To get along with my friend,

I check my friend's face to see what he is communicating.

Consider these situations.

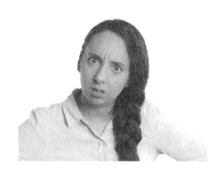

Katie is busy playing a game with Lisa, but she forgets to look at Lisa's face.

What information did she miss?

_____

What problem might that cause?

_____

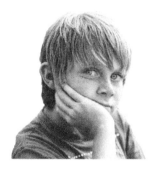

Liam saw this expression on Kasen's face after they'd been playing Mario for a while.

What is Kasen communicating?

_____

What can Liam do in this situation?

_____

2.6 Coaching Guide: Avoid being a space invader

Quick Reference:

> » Review the last worksheet

> » Introduce the Key Idea: Read, paraphrase, connect

> » Complete & review the worksheet

> » Extra practice

> » Revisit the Key Idea

> » Congratulate your learner & finish

General Notes: Children with Autism may be less aware of personal space and what is appropriate for hugging, holding hands, etc.

Since what is acceptable depends greatly on age and cultural norms, we don't give specific requirements in the following worksheet. We leave it to you to communicate with your learner about the cultural norms for their age and situation.

Extra Practice: If it is challenging for your learner to adjust from previously learned rules, consider preparing your learner for what is coming in a year or two. For example, in some cultures, older boys avoid holding hands with each other. If your young male learner is a hand-holder with his peers, you may want to start drawing his attention to how older boys act with each other.

Make sure any sensory needs can be met in other ways.

Your Notes/Extra Ideas:

2.6 Avoid being a space invader

To get along with my friend,

I avoid being a space invader.

Being a space invader is when you go into someone's personal space and it makes them feel uncomfortable.

Show/Tell your coach what is okay and not okay in each of these situations.

Playing tag

Sitting on a bench with a friend

Sitting on a bench with a stranger

Having a conversation

Walking together

Taking your friend to show them something

Giving something to a

Looking at the same book

Lying down on the grass

2.7 Coaching Guide: Make decisions together

Quick Reference:

> » Review the last worksheet
>
> » Introduce the Key Idea: Read, paraphrase, connect
>
> » Complete & review the worksheet
>
> » Extra practice
>
> » Revisit the Key Idea

General Notes: This worksheet focuses on an important part of friendship: making decisions together. To show friendship, you make decisions that suit the two of you, not just what suits yourself. This often involves compromise - the subject of the next worksheet.

Extra Practice: Role-play relevant situations from your student's daily life. Perhaps your learner needs to practice choosing a game with his brother, deciding what to do at recess, etc.

Your Notes/Extra Ideas:

2.7 Make decisions together

Friends make decisions together.

Which situation shows friends making decisions together?

At the food court at the mall.

Jill: What sort of food do you feel like?

Mia: What about Mexican?

Jill: Yeah. I really feel like tacos.

How does everyone feel after the decision is made?

_____

_____

On the playground.

Griff: Let's play soccer.

Hal: No. I want to play four-square.

Griff: We played that yesterday. Can we do soccer today?

Hal: No. I'm going to play four-square.

How does everyone feel after the decision is made?

_____

_____

2.8 Coaching Guide: Compromise

Quick Reference:

» Review the last worksheet

» Introduce the Key Idea: Read, paraphrase, connect

» Complete & review the worksheet

» Extra practice

» Revisit the Key Idea

» Congratulate your learner & finish

General Notes: Making decisions together (the previous worksheet) and playing together often involve compromising. Use this worksheet to give your learner practice in compromising. Make sure to discuss WHY compromising is a good idea.

Consider also, if you have a situation where your learner always compromises. In this case, your learner may need to build skills in communicating/asserting what they want.

Extra Practice: Use this opportunity to make sure your learner has compromising skills across the complete range of activities that he or she is likely to encounter.

Make sure to include video games, as they are an important part of child culture. Some children may find it very challenging to switch from solo play to playing with a friend. Evaluate and if necessary, build your learner's skills at compromising when playing video games with a peer.

Your Notes/Extra Ideas:

2.8 Compromise

When I play with my friend,

I compromise to find something that suits us both.

Think about the following situations and answer the questions.

Kiera always insists on going first when she plays a game.

How might her friends feel about this?_____

Why is that a problem?_____

_____

Dominic always wants to play soccer at lunchtime. Sometimes his friend Alex would rather play basketball.

What should they each do?_____

_____

Lucas likes to sprint ahead when he plays Mario, but Isaac likes to go slow and collect all the coins. When they play together, they often get mad at each other.

Why is getting mad a problem?_____

What can they do instead?_____

_____

2.9 Coaching Guide: Not my choice

Quick Reference:

» Review the last worksheet

» Introduce the Key Idea: Read, paraphrase, connect

» Complete & review the worksheet

» Extra practice

» Revisit the Key Idea

» Congratulate your learner & finish

General Notes: With compromising comes the likelihood that your learner will have to play a game that is not his/her preferred choice. In this worksheet, your student learns that it is important to do this graciously.

Extra Practice: Role-play situations directly related to your student's life. Include what you know about his preferences to make it more realistic.

Your Notes/Extra Ideas:

2.9 Not my choice

I enjoy the game, even if it is not my choice.

To show that we are a friend, we sometimes have to go along with our friend's choice of game or activity. We can do that happily or grumpily. Which do you think is best? Why?

Erin wants to play Shopkins. Her friend Layla gives an exasperated sigh and says, "Okay. If we have to."

How is each girl probably feeling now?_____

What is each girl probably thinking about the other?_____

_____

Is this good for their friendship? Why or why not?_____

_____

What would be a better outcome?_____

Tom agreed to play Transformers, but he isn't enjoying it much. He is feeling angry that he agreed to play. He is acting grumpy and rude.

How is Tom's friend probably feeling?_____

How might this affect their friendship?_____

_____

2.10 Coaching Guide: *Be a good sport*

Quick Reference:

> » Review the last worksheet
>
> » Introduce the Key Idea: Read, paraphrase, connect
>
> » Complete & review the worksheet
>
> » Extra practice
>
> » Revisit the Key Idea
>
> » Congratulate your learner & finish

General Notes: Another key skill for maintaining friendship is being able to lose graciously.

Extra Practice: As part of the learning for this topic, play games with your learner to see how skilled he or she is at losing gracefully.

Keep in mind that your learner may find it easier to lose some games than others. Losing at video games, for example, can be a real challenge for some learners. If needed, take this opportunity to help your learner build this skill.

Your Notes/Extra Ideas:

2.10 Be a good sport

If I lose a game, I am a good sport about it.

Losing is hard. But part of being a friend is being cool with losing so that your friend can enjoy winning.

Natalie is playing cards with Sofia. Natalie can see she is about to lose, so she throws her cards on the floor and walks away.

What do you think Sofia is thinking about Natalie?_____

How might this affect their friendship?_____

Joe always wins Monopoly when he plays with his sister. But today he lost. He is really mad at himself. He does his best to smile at his sister and say, "Good game."

How will his sister feel about that?_____

Will his sister want to play Monopoly with Joe again?_____

It's a rainy day and Kian is playing checkers with Mattias. Kian wins and Mattias is really disappointed. Afterwards, Mattias tells his other friends that Kian cheated.

Is Mattias being a good sport?_____

How do you think Kian will feel about Mattias if he hears what Mattias said?

_____

What is the right thing for Mattias to do now?_____

2.11 Coaching Guide: Friends share

Quick Reference:

» Review the last worksheet

» Introduce the Key Idea: Read, paraphrase, connect

» Complete & review the worksheet

» Extra practice

» Revisit the Key Idea

» Congratulate your learner & finish

General Notes: Sharing builds friendships, so use this opportunity to make sure your learner has this skill.

However, ensure your learner isn't always sharing without reciprocation. Our learners are easily taken advantage of.

Extra Practice: As always, consider YOUR student. What situations make sharing a challenge for your student? Is it food, favorite toys? Role-play challenging situations until you are confident your student can demonstrate appropriate responses.

Your Notes/Extra Ideas:

2.11 Friends share

If I bring out something fun to eat or do, I should share.

Sharing helps build friendships. Consider each of these situations and how it builds or weakens the friendship.

Jax and Alan are playing at Jax's house. Jax brings out a toy roller coaster and starts playing with it. He tells Alan that he can't play with it because it is too expensive.

How might Alan feel?_____

What should Jax do instead?_____

Peter and Milo are walking home from school. Peter buys some candy at the corner store, but Milo doesn't have any money. Peter gives some of his candy to Milo.

How might Milo feel about Peter's actions?_____

How might this affect their friendship?_____

Grace and Emily go to the movies. Grace buys an extra-large popcorn and during the movie she eats it all without offering any to Emily.

What might Emily be thinking?_____

How might that affect their friendship?_____

What could Grace have done differently?_____

Chapter 3
When Things Go Wrong

Friends are fun to be with, but sometimes you might get mad or frustrated with your friend. That's okay. It happens in every friendship. In this chapter, you will learn some ideas for getting your friendship back on track.

3.1 Coaching Guide: Consider my own behavior

Quick Reference:

> » Review the last worksheet

> » Introduce the Key Idea: Read, paraphrase, connect

> » Complete & review the worksheet

> » Extra practice

> » Revisit the Key Idea

General Notes: Some children take a while to learn that even though they themselves are enjoying something, it doesn't mean that their friend is enjoying it as well. In fact, it might be bothering or irritating their friend. This worksheet helps learners consider other people's perspectives.

Extra Practice: Where possible, discuss instances from your learner's experiences, especially if there is a pattern of behavior that is irritating to peers. The behavior might be quite innocent, but still prove irritating.

For example, one of my learners liked to play with people's names. He would say 'Ivan Shmivan' instead of 'Ivan'. This proved VERY irritating to some peers, and humorous to others. This student needed to learn that he had to stop playing with names when he was around peers who found it irritating.

Your Notes/Extra Ideas:

3.1 Consider my own behavior

If my friend is annoyed with me,

I stop doing things that bother my friend.

Consider these situations.

James like to rhyme his friends' names. His friend Latham thinks it is really funny. His friend Rob gets mad when James does it.

When they met to walk to school today, James said, "Hey, Rob Nob.'

How do you think Rob felt when James said this?_____

Will Rob want to hang out with James if he continues to do this?_____

What does James need to do instead? Why? _____

_____

Lara watches a lot of prank videos on YouTube. She often tries out the pranks on her friends and she thinks it is really funny. Her friends get mad with her because they don't like it.

Lara just watched a new prank video, and she is thinking of trying it on Monday.

How is Lara feeling about the prank video? _____

How will her friends feel if she pranks them again?_____

How might this affect their feelings about Lara?_____

_____

3.2 Coaching Guide: Apologize if needed

Quick Reference:

>> Review the last worksheet

>> Introduce the Key Idea: Read, paraphrase, connect

>> Complete & review the worksheet

>> Extra practice

>> Revisit the Key Idea

General Notes: Apologies can get friendships back on track quickly. Use this worksheet as an opportunity to make sure that your learner can do a quick, appropriate apology. Watch out for learners who apologize too much, as this can also be alienating for peers.

Extra Practice: Brainstorm some apology-needing situations with your learner and role-play appropriate responses.

Your Notes/Extra Ideas:

3.2 Apologize if needed

If my friend is annoyed with me,

I apologize if I have done something wrong.

Apologies should be quick and appropriate to the situation. After an apology, it is time to move on. Practice giving apologies for the following situations.

- Sheila bumps into a classmate as she is walking down the hall.
- Larson spills some of his drink on his best friend.

Now consider these situations.

Gina threw a ball that hit her friend Larissa in the head. Here's what happened next.

Gina: "I'm so sorry."

Larissa: "It's okay."

Gina: "But I'm really, really sorry."

Larissa: "I said it's okay."

Gina: "I'm really sorry."

What is the problem?_____

Fiona bumped Jeevan's arm as he was finishing an important drawing. When She noticed, she said "Oops."

Jeevan is feeling really mad.

What is the problem?_____

3.3 Coaching Guide: State my problem

Quick Reference:

» Review the last worksheet

» Introduce the Key Idea: Read, paraphrase, connect

» Complete & review the worksheet

» Extra practice

» Revisit the Key Idea

General Notes: The purpose of this worksheet is to help your learner know what to do if they are bothered by someone else's actions.

Take as much time as needed to make sure that your student learns to deliver their concerns in a **strong** voice and not an **upset** voice. A strong voice will serve them well as they get older. An upset voice becomes more and more inappropriate as they age beyond childhood.

Extra Practice: As always, practice as many examples as possible from your learner's experiences.

Your Notes/Extra Ideas:

3.3 State my problem

If I am annoyed with my friend,

I speak calmly and tell him what is bothering me.

A calm, strong voice gets better results than an upset or whiny voice. Use a strong, calm voice when you want people's actions to change.

Imagine you are in the following situations and practice giving a response in a strong, calm voice.

Your mom promised that you could choose the restaurant for the next family dinner. Now she says that it's your brother's turn to choose. This is a big deal for you.

How will you respond to your mother?

_____

Your classmate won't give your iPhone back. You are really mad because you think you might miss the bus if you don't leave now.

How will you respond to your classmate?

_____

Your brother keeps poking you, even though you've asked him to stop.

How will you respond to your brother?

_____

3.4 Coaching Guide: Choose something else

Quick Reference:

> » Review the last worksheet

> » Introduce the Key Idea: Read, paraphrase, connect

> » Complete & review the worksheet

> » Extra practice

> » Revisit the Key Idea

General Notes: In this worksheet, your student learns that it is okay to remove himself from a situation if it is bothersome. This could mean moving just a few inches away, or completely removing himself from the situation if that is more appropriate.

Extra Practice: Your learner will be the best resource for identifying situations where his friends have frustrated him. Role-play using the 'moving away' strategy as a solution. Talk about when it would work and when it would not... and what to do in that situation.

Your Notes/Extra Ideas:

3.4 Choose something else

If my friend continues to bother me,

I move away and do something else.

Consider these situations and choose what to do.

Carla is in her neighbor Eva's yard with her friend Eva. Eva is jumping on a pogo stick and won't give Carla a turn, even though she's asked several times. Carla is getting really annoyed.

What could Carla do?_____

_____

Felip's friend Max is in a bad mood and keeps kicking Felip's chair during lunch. Felip has asked Max to stop, but he doesn't.

What could Felip do if Max doesn't listen to him?_____

_____

George wants to play catch with his friend Leo, but Leo keeps throwing the ball so hard that George can't catch it. George has asked Leo to throw the ball more softly, but Leo is still throwing it really hard.

What could George do if Leo doesn't listen to him?_____

_____

3.5 Coaching Guide: Accept other's opinions

Quick Reference:

» Review the last worksheet

» Introduce the Key Idea: Read, paraphrase, connect

» Complete & review the worksheet

» Extra practice

» Revisit the Key Idea

General Notes: ASD learners often need support in learning that other people have different opinions... and that this is okay. This worksheet helps your learner practice what to say if their friend does not agree with them.

Extra Practice: Ask your learner about situations where he/she has had an argument with a friend. Role-play different ways of dealing with the situation. Talk about the pros and cons of each approach.

Your Notes/Extra Ideas:

3.5 Accept other's opinions

If my friend and I argue,

I accept that others may have different opinions.

Consider these situations.

Hal and Greta are talking about their favorite movies. Hal loves Star Wars, but Greta thinks they are a waste of time.

What would you say if you were Hal?

_____

_____

Reed knows the next baseball game is on Saturday, but Kian is adamant that the game is on Sunday.

What would you say if you were Reed?

_____

_____

Shay thinks that Marie agreed to go to the movies with her. Marie is pretty sure she never said that.

What would you say if you were Marie?

_____

_____

3.6 Coaching Guide: Cool down

Quick Reference:

>> Review the last worksheet

>> Introduce the Key Idea: Read, paraphrase, connect

>> Complete & review the worksheet

>> Extra practice

>> Revisit the Key Idea

>> Congratulate your learner & finish

General Notes: When we are upset, our emotions rule our actions. If we cool down, the logical part of our brain gets a chance to get involved. This worksheet helps learners understand that it is okay to take time to cool down.

Extra Practice: Talk through/role-play situations from your student's life where he/she was really upset about something.

Your Notes/Extra Ideas:

3.6 Cool down

If I get really upset with my friend,

I give myself space to cool down.

Consider these situations.

Jason and Regan are arguing over who lost the school soccer ball. Jason is getting angrier and angrier because he knows Regan lost the ball.

If Regan won't listen to him, what could Jason do to cool down?

_____

_____

Lisa's mom is blaming her for eating all the ice cream. Lisa only ate a little bit of ice cream and she is really mad that her mom won't listen to her.

What can Lisa do to cool down?

_____

_____

Adrian just discovered that his little brother destroyed the school assignment Adrian had been working on for a week. He is feeling really mad and wants to go confront his brother.

Should Adrian go confront his brother now? What else could he do?

_____

_____

3.7 Coaching Guide: No hard feelings

Quick Reference:

> » Review the last worksheet
>
> » Introduce the Key Idea: Read, paraphrase, connect
>
> » Complete & review the worksheet
>
> » Extra practice
>
> » Revisit the Key Idea
>
> » Congratulate your learner & finish

General Notes: Holding a grudge does not build a friendship. With this lesson, ensure that your learner knows how to act/react the next time he encounters a friend he has had a disagreement with.

Extra Practice: Ask for examples from your student's life where he has reacted appropriately or not appropriately after an argument or disagreement. Role-play alternate reactions.

Your Notes/Extra Ideas:

3.7 No hard feelings

If we have an argument,

next time I see my friend I smile and say 'Hi' to show

there are no hard feelings.

Consider these situations.

Kyla and Tara had a disagreement at lunchtime about which lunch club to go to. They ended up going to separate clubs. They see each other after lunch.

What is a good way to show there are no hard feelings?

_____

_____

Oliver is mad at Reno for losing his basketball. Reno replaces the ball and gives it to Oliver at school.

What is a good way for Oliver to show there are no hard feelings?

_____

_____

Jason's dad drank the chocolate milk that Jason bought with his own money. Jason is mad because he was looking forward to drinking it after his baseball game.

How should each react to this situation?

_____

_____

Chapter 4 Challenging Situations

Sometimes your friend might suggest that you do something that is wrong. It's important to know how to react in these types of situations so that you make good choices.

In this chapter, you will practice responding in situations where you must choose the right thing to do.

4.1 Coaching Guide: Saying no

Quick Reference:

» Review the last worksheet

» Introduce the Key Idea: Read, paraphrase, connect

» Complete & review the worksheet

» Extra practice

» Revisit the Key Idea

General Notes: It is really important that our students know how to say no. In much of their lives, compliance is rewarded. So for challenging situations, we need to make sure that they have the ability to identify an inappropriate situation and also the ability to say no to it.

Extra Practice: Practice with situations that are likely to occur in your learner's life. Don't forget to ask your learner for ideas of challenging situations he has experienced or knows about.

Your Notes/Extra Ideas:

4.1 Saying no

If my friend suggests something that I think is wrong,

I say no in a calm, strong voice. I don't need to explain myself.

Consider these situations.

Your friend wants to ring the doorbell on a neighbor's house and then run away.

What will you say?

_____

Your friend asks if he can copy your math homework because he forgot to do his.

What will you say?

_____

Your friend shows you a packet of cigarettes and offers you one.

What will you say?

_____

A friend wants you to come with him while he shoplifts some candy.

What will you say?

_____

4.2 Suggest an alternative

Quick Reference:

>> Review the last worksheet

>> Introduce the Key Idea: Read, paraphrase, connect

>> Complete & review the worksheet

>> Extra practice

>> Revisit the Key Idea

>> Congratulate your learner & finish

General Notes: The purpose of this worksheet is to help your learner know what to do next in a situation where his peer is encouraging inappropriate behavior. The first step is to say no (the previous worksheet), the next step is to encourage his friend to move on to something more appropriate.

Extra Practice: Use additional examples from your learner's everyday experiences.

Your Notes/Extra Ideas:

4.2 Suggest an alternative

If my friend suggests something that I think is wrong,

I suggest something else to do.

Consider each of the following situations.

You are walking home from school and your friend suggests you both investigate a building site, even though it has big signs saying 'No trespassing.'

What will you say? What else can you suggest?

_____

_____

You and your friend have just finished watching a movie at the big Cineplex. Your friend suggests you both sneak into another cinema to see another movie for free.

What will you say? What else can you suggest?

_____

_____

Your mom has told you that you aren't allowed to play on the treadmill. Your friend suggests you both get on and make it go really fast.

What will you say? What else can you suggest?

_____

_____

4.3 Coaching Guide: Walk away

Quick Reference:

» Review the last worksheet

» Introduce the Key Idea: Read, paraphrase, connect

» Complete & review the worksheet

» Extra practice

» Revisit the Key Idea

» Congratulate your learner & finish

General Notes: The purpose of this worksheet is to let your learner know that it is okay to walk away from a situation. We can't always influence our friend's choices, so sometimes walking away is the best option.

Extra Practice: Ask your learner for similar situations from their own life.

Your Notes/Extra Ideas:

4.3 Walk away

If my friend suggests something that I think is wrong,

I can walk away.

Consider each of these situations.

Your friend wants to draw some graffiti in an alley near your house. He has some spray paint and wants you to help.

What will you say and do?

_____

_____

You and your friend are at his house. Your friend starts watching a video on YouTube that you know your mom wouldn't want you watching.

What will you say and do?

_____

_____

You are at the pool with your friend and he tries to break into the vending machine to get a free can of drink.

What will you say and do?

_____

_____

4.4 Coaching Guide: Talk to an adult

Quick Reference:

>> Review the last worksheet

>> Introduce the Key Idea: Read, paraphrase, connect

>> Complete & review the worksheet

>> Extra practice

>> Revisit the Key Idea

>> Congratulate your learner & finish

General Notes: Children who face challenging situations need to know that they can talk to a trusted adult. While we may think that children know this already, it is important to reinforce this idea regularly.

Extra Practice: Ask your learner for situations from his/her own experiences which have been challenging to deal with. As always, discussions based in actual experiences will have more meaning for our learners.

Your Notes/Extra Ideas:

4.4 Talk to an adult

If my friend often suggests things that I think are wrong,

I can talk to my mom or dad or a trusted adult to get their opinion.

Consider these situations.

Your friend Lisa has been video-chatting with a stranger online and she wants you to join in. You've told her that you think talking with a stranger is a bad idea, but she just laughs and doesn't listen to you. She's asked you to keep this a secret.

What could you do? _____

_____

One of your friends has been shoplifting candy on the weekends. He's started doing it while you are with him. You told him to stop but he ignores you. You are worried that you will be caught with him, even though you haven't ever taken anything.

What could you do? _____

_____

Your friend Kerry sometimes asks you to lie to her parents and say that she was at your place. You don't like lying, but Kerry keeps asking you to do it.

What could you do? _____

_____

4.5 Coaching Guide: *False friends*

Quick Reference:

> » Review the last worksheet

> » Introduce the Key Idea: Read, paraphrase, connect

> » Complete & review the worksheet

> » Extra practice

> » Revisit the Key Idea

> » Congratulate your learner & finish

General Notes: Children with Autism need to know about false friends. Because of their underdeveloped social skills, ASD students can be easy targets for mean kids and bullies. Use this worksheet to help your learner differentiate between real friends and false friends. You can also refer back to the criteria in Chapter 1, which identified how real friends act.

Encourage your learner to walk away from false friends and to discuss the situation with a trusted adult.

Extra Practice: Ask your learner for situations that he or she has experienced to help him/her put these skills into practice.

Your Notes/Extra Ideas:

4.5 False friends

I should watch out for false friends. False friends:

- say mean things to you or about you to other people

- encourage you to do or say bad things

- laugh at you when you don't want them to

- pretend to include you, but really exclude you

Some people might pretend to be your friend, but they aren't really. Watch out for people who don't treat you like a friend should.

Don't spend time with false friends. Walk away and find something else to do.

Which of these situations might be false friends? What would you suggest Katie and Peter do?

Katie feels uncomfortable around Jackie and Sienna because they often make exaggerated comments about how great her hair looks. She thinks they might be laughing at her, but she's not sure.

Mike and Liam always invite Peter to play basketball at lunch, but they never pass the ball to him. They keep saying, "Here you go," but never actually throw the ball to him.

Chapter 5
Fun Things to do
with Friends

For the coach:

To finish the book on a positive note, in this chapter we put the emphasis back on good times with friends.

It is easy to assume that kids know what friends do together. But this can be an incorrect assumption for ASD learners. They may not actually know what to do with a friend. Or if they do know what type of thing to do, they may not be able to *do it* effectively.

The goal for this chapter is to ensure that your learner has the skills to actually engage in an activity with a friend.

This chapter deviates from the typical Six-Minute model. Instead of providing worksheets targeting a specific **social rule**, like in the rest of the workbook, this chapter provides you with assessments to evaluate your learner's current ability with specific **social activities**.

We include eight different types of activities that are important for children's social success. Feel free to add different categories to suit your needs. An extra checklist is included at the end for this purpose.

The activity skills we cover are:

1. Active Structured Play

This includes organized sports such as basketball and soccer, as well as more informal games such as four-square, hopscotch, etc. In these games there are a set of rules that stay fairly static.

2. Active Unstructured Play

This category includes games like roleplaying or pretend games, where there are no set rules ahead of time, but the 'rules' emerge as play unfolds. This category may also include games with known rules that get changed over time. For example, a game of tag where new rules are added during play.

There is not a clear line between structured an unstructured play. However, the more unstructured the play, the more likely it is to be challenging for our learners.

3. Board Games & Card Games

This category of activities includes board games and card games. Basically, any game that is structured but not particularly active.

4. Video Games

This popular category includes games on any type of screen. As children often play these games solo, you may need to have a specific focus on ensuring that they have the skills to play these games with a friend.

5. Making or Creating Things

This category of activities includes anything from Lego, to building paper airplanes, to painting/crafting, to making music, to constructing a fort in the backyard. If your learner is a builder or creator, then this can be a great first priority as activities can quite naturally be morphed from individual projects (parallel play) to group projects (cooperative play.)

6, 7 & 8: Conversion Skills

Talking is perhaps the most important skill for engaging with a friend. We include three specific talking skills in this section: comparing thoughts and opinions, talking about shared experiences, and making plans. A more thorough development of conversation skills can be found in Six-Minute Social Skills Workbook 1.

6. Conversation: Comparing Thoughts and Opinions

We might tell our students to talk to their friends, but we need to make sure that our learners know what to talk about. One common activity is comparing thoughts and opinions about favorite topics. This might be talking about the latest Star Wars movie, comparing sports teams, or pretty much anything your learner is interested in.

7. Conversation: Talking about Shared Experiences

Another excellent activity with friends is to talk about past experiences they have shared. This builds strong connections between kids.

8. Conversation: Make Plans Together

Friends do things together, so being able to make plans to do things together is an important skill. Depending on the age of your learner, appropriate ways to perform this skill may include in-person, phone call or text invitations.

Once you have evaluated your learner's play skills using the worksheets, consider where the weaknesses are. You will probably find a similar pattern of weaknesses across the different play types.

Next, determine how you will remediate these skills.

The following stages may help you progress from teaching the skill through to generalization.

1. Teach/build the skill in a structured environment with an adult.

2. Practice the skill in a natural environment with other adults who understand the learner's challenges.

3. Practice the skill with a familiar, flexible peer (perhaps a sibling?)

4. Provide light support in the natural environment with other peers. Remove support as soon as possible.

Good luck with building your learner's social activity skills. When combined with a strong understanding of the social rules of friendship, your learner will become unstoppable!!

5.1 Activity Evaluation: Active Structured Play

Can your student independently initiate various types of active structured play with a peer?

Can your student independently organize from the idea of play through to play starting?

Does your student maintain emotional regulation throughout the play?

Does your student communicate appropriately throughout the play?

- appropriately initiates communication
- appropriately responds to communication
- appropriately continues communication

Does your student appropriately maintain attention throughout the play, noticing things like whose turn, when the rules change, etc?

5.1 Activity Evaluation continued: Active Structured Play

Does your student exhibit cooperation and compromise appropriately throughout the play? (This includes taking turns, following the rules, etc.)

Does your learner handle the situation when things go badly?

Can your learner exit play appropriately, either at the end of the game or when they want to stop?

What specific types of active structured play do your student's peers do regularly?

How important is this type of play for fitting in with your learner's peers?

Additional Notes:

5.2 Activity Evaluation: Active Unstructured Play

Can your student independently initiate various types of active unstructured play with a peer?

Can your student independently organize from the idea of play through to play starting?

Does your student maintain emotional regulation throughout the play?

Does your student communicate appropriately throughout the play?

- appropriately initiates communication

- appropriately responds to communication

- appropriately continues communication

Does your student appropriately maintain attention throughout the play, noticing things like whose turn, when the rules change, etc?

5.2 Activity Evaluation Continued: Active Unstructured Play

Does your student exhibit cooperation and compromise appropriately throughout the play? (This includes taking turns, following the rules, etc.)

Does your learner handle the situation when things go badly?

Can your learner exit play appropriately, either at the end of the game or when they want to stop?

Does your student add his/her own ideas to the play? Are they appropriate to the situation?

How important is this type of play for fitting in with your learner's peers?

Additional Notes:

5.3 Activity Evaluation: Board Games & Card Games

Can your student independently initiate various examples of this type of play with a peer?

_____

_____

Can your student independently organize from the idea of play through to play starting?

_____

_____

Does your student maintain emotional regulation throughout the play?

_____

_____

Does your student communicate appropriately throughout the play?

- appropriately initiates communication
- appropriately responds to communication
- appropriately continues communication

_____

_____

Does your student appropriately maintain attention throughout the play, noticing things like whose turn, when the rules change, etc?

_____

_____

5.3 Activity Evaluation Continued: Board Games & Card Games

Does your student exhibit cooperation and compromise appropriately throughout the play? (This includes taking turns, following the rules, etc.)

Does your learner handle the situation when things go badly?

Can your learner exit play appropriately, either at the end of the game or when they want to stop?

What types of board games and card games do your student's peers play?

How important is this type of play for fitting in with your learner's peers?

Additional Notes:

5.4 Activity Evaluation: Video Games

Can your student independently initiate playing various video games with a peer?

_____

_____

Can your student independently organize from the idea of play through to play starting?

_____

_____

Does your student maintain emotional regulation throughout the play?

_____

_____

Does your student communicate appropriately throughout the play?

- appropriately initiates communication
- appropriately responds to communication
- appropriately continues communication

_____

_____

Does your student appropriately maintain attention throughout the play, noticing things like whose turn, when the rules change, etc?

_____

_____

5.4 Activity Evaluation Continued: Video Games

Does your student exhibit cooperation and compromise appropriately throughout the play? (This includes taking turns, following the rules, etc.)

Does your learner handle the situation when things go badly?

Can your learner exit play appropriately, either at the end of the game or when they want to stop?

What video games do your learner's peers play? Can your student play these games proficiently enough?

How important is this type of play for fitting in with your learner's peers?

Additional Notes:

5.5 Activity Evaluation: Building & Creating

Can your student independently initiate various examples of this type of play with a peer?

_____

_____

Can your student independently organize from the idea of play through to play starting?

_____

_____

Does your student maintain emotional regulation throughout the play?

_____

_____

Does your student communicate appropriately throughout the play?

- appropriately initiates communication

- appropriately responds to communication

- appropriately continues communication

_____

_____

Does your student appropriately maintain attention throughout the play, noticing things like whose turn, when the rules change, etc?

_____

_____

5.5 Activity Evaluation Continued: Building & Creating

Does your student exhibit cooperation and compromise appropriately throughout the play? (This includes taking turns, following the rules, etc.)

Does your learner handle the situation when things go badly?

Can your learner exit play appropriately, either at the end of the game or when they want to stop?

Does your student add his/her own ideas? Are they appropriate to the situation?

How important is this type of play for fitting in with your learner's peers?

Additional Notes:

5.6 Activity Evaluation: Comparing Thoughts & Opinions

Can your student independently initiate this type of conversation on a wide variety of topics?

Does your student maintain emotional regulation throughout the conversation?

Does your student successfully:

- initiate communication?

- respond?

- ask follow-up questions?

Does your student appropriately maintain attention throughout the conversation?

Does your student appropriately stay on topic during the conversation?

5.7 Activity Evaluation Continued: Comparing Thoughts & Opinions

Does your learner handle the situation when disagreements happen?

_____

_____

Can your learner exit conversations appropriately?

_____

_____

Does your student add his/her own ideas? Are they appropriate to the conversation?

_____

_____

Additional Notes:

_____

_____

_____

_____

_____

_____

5.7 Activity Evaluation: Talking about Shared Experiences

Can your student independently initiate this type of conversation on a wide variety of experiences?

_____

_____

Does your student maintain emotional regulation throughout the conversation?

_____

_____

Does your student successfully:

- initiate communication?

- respond?

- ask follow-up questions?

_____

_____

Does your student appropriately maintain attention throughout the conversation?

_____

_____

Does your student appropriately stay on topic during the conversation?

_____

_____

5.7 Activity Evaluation Continued: Talking about Shared Experiences

Does your learner handle the situation when disagreements happen?

_____

_____

Can your learner exit conversations appropriately?

_____

_____

Does your student add his/her own ideas? Are they appropriate to the conversation?

_____

_____

Additional Notes:

_____

_____

_____

_____

_____

5.8 Activity Evaluation: Making Plans

Can your student independently initiate this type of conversation?

Can your student independently make plans with a peer? (includes deciding activity, time and location and getting relevant permissions from parents.)

Can your learner negotiate changes or adjustment to a plan with a peer?

How important is this type of conversation for fitting in with your learner's peers?

Additional Notes:

5.9 Activity Evaluation:

Can your student independently initiate this type of play?

Can your student independently organize from the idea of play through to play starting?

Does the student maintain emotional regulation throughout the play?

Does the student communicate appropriately throughout the play?

- appropriately initiates communication

- appropriately responds to communication

- appropriately continues communication

Does the student appropriately maintain attention throughout the play, noticing things like whose turn, when the rules change, etc?

5.9 Activity Checklist Evaluation:

Does the student exhibit cooperation and compromise appropriately throughout the play? (This includes taking turns, following the rules, etc.)

Does your learner handle the situation when things go badly?

Can your learner exit play appropriately, either at the end of the game or when they want to stop?

Unstructured activities: Did your student add his/her own ideas? Were they appropriate to the situation?

How important is this type of play for fitting in with your learner's peers?

Additional Notes:

What Next?

Check out the other books in our Six-Minute Social Skills series! Although numbered, these books can be used in any order.

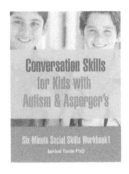 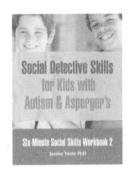

Available on Amazon or at
http://www.happyfroglearning.com/

These books build social confidence in quick easy steps. Grab them today in print or Kindle.

Key Ideas Summary

Download a one-page summary of all the Key Ideas introduced in the workbook. Great for quick reference!

Available for free on our website:

www.HappyFrogLearning.com/Friendship-Skills-PDF

Need More Resources?

www.HappyFrogLearning.com

Happy Frog Learning creates quality resources for children and teens with autism and other social/language challenges.

Our award-winning apps, workbooks and curriculums target reading comprehension, social skills and writing.

CERTIFICATE
OF
ACHIEVEMENT

THIS CERTIFICATE IS AWARDED TO

_____

IN RECOGNITION OF

_____

_____   _____

DATE   SIGNATURE

Made in the USA
Middletown, DE
09 March 2024

51149011R00064